THE MUSICIAN'S GUIDE TO SURVIVING THE ROCK STAR LIFESTYLE

This literature is based largely off of my experience and opinion. All bias is mine. I take full credit and responsibility. Where facts are given, you'll see the scholarly sources listed. Other than that, don't get all bent out of shape if you happen to disagree. It's cool. You're allowed to. These words are a stepping stone to help show people that health and wellness isn't terrifying. The smallest actions have the greatest reward. The words of this book are coached, written, spoken, influenced, played and created by me, Mike Schwartz. I'll own that shit.

Embrace change. Become a better human.

You're somebody's superhero.

Created, Written & Handcrafted by Mike Schwartz

All Rights Reserved

Cover photo copyright Tyler Branston 2017. Image of Mike Sands of All Else Fails performing in Surrey, BC in 2011. Image used under license from Tyler Branston, with permission from Mike Sands and All Else Fails.

Foreword by Lisa Anderson

Edited by Tanner James

Back photo copyright Sean Schwartz Photography©

ISBN 978-1-365-70718-6

For more information on Mike Schwartz' vibe, services, and his mission to bring health & wellness to the forefront of the music industry please visit www.mikeschwartz.ca

Published by PPLSKLZ©

Check the Podcast. We're on iTunes! PPLSKLZ RADIO

You don't have to be a rock star to start.

You just have to start in order to become a rock star.

Table Of Contents

For my Omi & Opa. Thank you for showing me what it is to give the greatest love, unconditionally. Opa, you were right. Not quite a politician...yet. I'm just bettering myself everyday and I help others do the same. I hope this book takes it one step further.

Dankeshön. Ich liebe dich.

For those of us just trying to find our place, tell our story and bring the love...
Don't wait for it to happen. Make it happen. Thanks pops.

Foreword

Growing up in a very active family, I was lucky to have healthy exercise and eating regimes implemented in my daily routine from a young age. However, when I moved out on my own and got more into the music scene, some of those habits proved difficult to maintain.

Like so many musicians, the late nights and long practice sessions began to wear on my body. I struggled to have enough energy and stamina to continue working at the fast pace this industry requires. I woke up sore every day, and was going to physiotherapy for tendonitis in both wrists. I knew that exercising would give me more energy and that strengthening my muscles would reduce the everyday strains caused by playing, but I didn't really know where to start.

Fortuitously, I met Mike at a show we were both playing and found out about his fitness endeavours. He briefly told me about his restorative approach, and I couldn't wait to start training with him. He's given me so many great tools that have improved my well-being, and their effects have trickled down to every facet of my life. I am happier, more energized, and more creative. It's essentially helped transform me into a better version of myself.

I know that if I want any sort of longevity in this business I need to take good care of my body, mind, and soul, and when one is lacking the others follow suit. Like anything, fitness requires effort, but that's where Mike and this book can help. They'll give you a plan to follow, and they'll keep you accountable. If you stick with it, you will feel the results. You'll get what you give tenfold, and trust me, you're worth it!

- Lisa Anderson, Singer/Songwriter, Calgary, Alberta

Preface
The first thing I want you to know is that I don't know anything…

That's right, nothing. I learned this back in 2012 during my C.H.E.K Holistic Lifestyle Certification down in San Francisco. The gentleman instructing the course, JP Sears (shout out to JP who has done some really amazing things in the industry) challenged the class to remove all ego from any given situation in order to better understand another perspective. It may not have made sense to me then, but it sure does now. Go figure, if you know nothing about any given topic, you're surely going to learn something. And that's been my approach ever since. Learn from every thing, everyone, and every situation. I believe there is no such thing as a mistake. Only experience.

That said, when I set out to write this book it was my goal to take what I have learned over the years and try my best to communicate it to my peers in the music industry. It took me quite some time to blend my passion for music with well, let's call it *wellness.* Movement, nutrition and mindset really - the three pillars that shape the foundation of my coaching philosophy. I still hear JP's words back in Frisco ringing in my head whenever I come across another trainer or coach with a different approach from mine. I try to remove my beliefs (and it's hard at times), but I believe I have achieved my level of success in the industry partially due to keeping my mouth shut and my ego in check. It was a struggle at times as I'm a pretty opinionated guy… so if this sounds like you, I'd encourage you to do the same. You may find that you tend to learn more when you *don't know anything at all.*

So now you know where I'm coming from at least. Now, what's this book all about? What are you in for? Well little missy, let me tell you…! This is an accumulation of my combined ten years or so of music industry and fitness industry experience. I have been playing drums in the local Calgary scene since I was 18. I have been a certified personal trainer for nearly ten years. I have seen a lot in both worlds and have now taken the opportunity to blend my passions of music and fitness. Funny enough, when I describe what I do to anyone, I get the same reaction. Typically the person looks at me like I have three heads and says something to the effect of "What? You're crazy! Musicians can't afford training… you're wasting your time." Well, thank you sir or madame, but I come from the school that when you show value, cost is irrelevant. Musicians are people too, no different than the next profession. Actually, perhaps that's the root of it. Maybe musicians need to start treating themselves as professionals, like lawyers or business executives in some sense. Maybe our health would follow suit, if we followed the suits a bit…

In my experience, the stigma of musicians and health is largely blown out of proportion. It's not that we don't want to live a healthy life. Rather, it's a matter of the industry not having the knowledge, support or skills to start taking a closer look at health, performance and career longevity. I am incredibly passionate about helping people. I am also incredibly passionate about music. Not just as a creator, performer or artist myself, but also as a listener. I would like to continue to hear amazing music for as long as I live, so if I can help keep an artist on the road, managing - not removing - the consequences of the lifestyle, I feel as though I have done my part for the betterment of society. I'm sure if you love great music, you'll agree. The feeling I get when I know I have had a hand in helping another person achieve what they were told they wouldn't or when I know I have passed on skills that another person can pay forward, and then that person pays it forward again and again… that's what I live for. So for me, it's a no brainer to bring my attention to the music industry. This is a passion project and within the next eighty pages or so I hope to have educated, inspired or somehow changed for the better, your perspective on health, performance and overall quality of life.

While what I write on these pages is founded in science and backed up in experience, I can't stress enough that this book is not an absolute. I have a hard time with any sort of absolutes. This is simply a collection of what I have seen, what I have done and what's worked for me in the past. By no means should any of my theory be taken as "the word". I encourage you to read, educate yourself and then apply to practice. We are all individuals and my experience may very well be different than yours. Might work, might not. But I do guarantee one thing: the fact that you picked up this book signifies you're ready to make a change and that, my friend, is half the battle! It may not be exactly the methods of exercise or the meal plans I've enclosed here that do it for you, but you'll find your way because you're ready to find your way. So feel good about that; congratulations! I am right here with you. I oftentimes tell folks with whom I'm privileged to work, that it can be a big, thick, nasty part of the woods we're lost in. But heck, it's better to be lost together, right? Keep in mind, I'm not trying to remove these little bits of lifestyle. Just simply trying to manage them so you can last a little longer at the party. Now let's get at it and get out of those woods! This is The Musician's Guide to Surviving the Rock Star Lifestyle and you are just pages away from learning how movement, nutrition and mindset can and will improve your performance, extend your career in the business, and ultimately increase your overall quality of life. You'll be better at everything, and I think that's the best thing that you can be. Unless you can be Batman. Then you should be Batman.

DISCLAIMER

The rest of this book is based on experience. While it's all factual, the first thing I learned in both the fitness and music industries is that there's more than one right way. When I talk about exercise and nutrition and mindset things, please discuss these things with a trusted health professional before undertaking it as "the word". I'm not going to be there to CPR your ass if you keel over or something, so be safe kids. Another note, you need to want this. You need to want to change. The topics I discuss in this book purely intrinsically motivated - meaning, in short, I can't do the push-ups for you. So please, if you're not quite ready to make some serious change put this book down and come back to it when you are. Furthermore, when you're done, do not hesitate to contact me and let me know what areas of your life you are working on and inspired to change. The reason I put this out there is to inspire change so, albeit a little selfishly, I wanna hear from you. Okay. Now that that's settled… Strap in, shit's about to get weird.

"People don't buy what you do; they buy why you do it. And what you do simply proves what you believe"

— *Simon Sinek, Start with Why: How Great Leaders Inspire Everyone to Take Action*

MY "WHY."

As a musician myself, I speak your language.

Let me set the stage: Intergalactic Lovers, Ampere, Munich, Germany, July 2015 -

Navigating the dark alleys and frenzied Bahn of Munich on a Friday night only speaking conversational German has its perks.

With 25kg on my back I happened to stumble upon the Ampere, a nightclub set deep near the river that happened to be host of the Belgian Indie rock group Intergalactic Lovers. This was a band I was stoked to see perform while I was in Germany. It was well past the opening band's set by the time I got to Munich, and I had no idea what direction was up. I was convinced that I was not going to make it. I pulled my iPhone out and sucked up the massive data bill I was going to face to get my bearings straight. At that moment, I just so happened to pass a guy wrapped up in a sheepskin poncho, let's call him Hank… and asked Hank "Sie wissen, wo das Ampere ist?" He pointed across the street towards a dark, enchanted forest.

This was my fate? Into what looked like a sure-fire deathbed full of hippies, the homeless and gangs? Really, Munich… Really?

I cowboy-ed up, slung my pack back on and trudged across the busy intersection into never-never-land. Sure enough, poncho-man was right, the Ampere was just off to the right. There was a dimly lit club sign and a few bigger guys outside lighting up their darts. After about 10 minutes of back and forth

"Germenglish" with the doorman, Gunther, I was let in to catch the last half of the Lovers' set, with the understanding that I would "be good to the bartender and buy beers..."

I was in, no line, no cover.

I watched the set and hung around to meet the Lovers. Hell, I was in Munich already and didn't have to be in Frankfurt for my flight home until about 10am. Nothing but time. I'll train overnight. After I met the gang, got my vinyl autographed and started talking to them about the tour, it all clicked. Maarten Huygens, the Lovers' guitarist was in bad shape. He had some severe shoulder and back pain - so much that the rest of the band asked me to go help him fix it. I was in my wheelhouse!

That night, instead of going to bed, I stuck around the grungy German club, showing Maarten how to stretch out his neck, wrists and shoulders. We stayed up 'til 4am working on little drills until I had to catch the train to Frankfurt. They all loved it. They asked me to come along on the road as their trainer. It all clicked. I thought: "I can help take care of bands so they can keep making the music we love."

I barely made my flight home. But I still have their vinyl and they still ask me how to fix Maarten, so that's rad. This is what I do. I don't get rid of the party, I just show you how to survive it. You don't have to be a rock star to start, you just have to start in order to become a rock star.

Part 1: Movement

Movement.

Chapter 1: The First Thing Every Musician Ever Needs To Do: Recognize The Problem

"All human beings should be able and willing to perform basic maintenance on themselves."

— *Kelly Starrett, Ready to Run: Unlocking Your Potential to Run Naturally*

I think the first time I realized I needed to do something was on the third night on tour with Matt Blais, in the summer of 2012. We were playing to a Stampede-esque festival in a big barn in the quiet logging community of Armstrong, British Columbia. We were hired for three forty-five minute sets, packed full of high energy blues rock and some classic cover tunes to keep the party going. That shit wears on you. The spot right between my shoulder blades was on fire, my hips were locking up and I'm pretty sure I stopped sweating - a sure sign of dehydration - after about the 4th song into the set. My mouth was dry, lips chapped and my body ached. We still had another hour to go. How the 'eff' was I going to get through the night?

Does this sound like you? Completely neglecting your body for the sake of the performance. Well, if it does, I'm telling you that you will want to stop that if you want any hope in hell of making a career out of this industry. Movement happens (or should happen) everyday. Proper movement... well that's another story. We as humans tend to cater to what is comfortable, and unfortunately, what's comfortable isn't always the proper movement patterning. So, when we're dealing with movement patterns that start to slip out of proper form, over time we build up imbalances and really shitty things start to happen to our bodies.

The first step is recognizing that you have a physical problem (ironically similar to the other Step Program that musicians find themselves getting into…). This could show itself in many ways, but injuries are the most dominant and annoying symptom so the next chapter will address the most common ones I have seen. You'll learn how to recognize the issue before it gets too far gone, so that's really cool too. Onward!

Chapter 2: The Common Areas of Every Musician's Body That Always Hurt, All Of The Time

Now, before you lead singers/rappers/vocalists, et al get all bent out of shape, know that I'm working on a second book tailored to you, because let's face it - you're kind of a big deal. A lot of the problems we see in the neck will resonate, but I know there's a lot of vocal warmups, therapy techniques that I still have to research more myself before writing about them. I don't yet have extensive therapeutic work with these musicians, but I am working hard to bring some relief to those that use the body as their main instrument. I appreciate your patience! Here's what I've got a real good handle on:

Shoulders and neck. Elbows and wrists. Lower back and hips.

There. Simple, right? Over the years these three zones have given more musicians more problems than a newbie sound guy in a dive bar. It's just plain ugly. Let's take a closer look at each particular area to get a feel for what causes problems for musicians. When assessing clients, I like to look at lifestyle issues like posture, stress, rest and fuel, as well as physical movement. Repetitive movements - more commonly poorly patterned repetitive movements - are major culprits of many, rather avoidable issues in all of these areas. Let's start from the top!

Shoulders and Neck

For every musician, the first areas I see a ton of problems in are the neck, shoulders and upper back (right between the shoulder blades). Why? Well it's pretty similar across the board. For drummers, just watch Dave Grohl in Nirvana's "Smells Like Teen

Spirit" music video. If the way he's setup bashing those tubs all hunched over and shit isn't a sure-fire way to neanderthal-like posture in a couple years, I don't know what is. And don't think you guitarists, strings, keys and even singers are off the hook on shitty postural habits... you're all pretty effin' terrible. Swinging your hair around and head banging doesn't help, as I'm sure you can imagine. Neither does leaving that bass way down past your knees and curling your spine like Quasimodo going to ring the bell... Meet our first reason every musician ever has shoulder and neck problems: hunched over, poor-as-shit posture. Fear not, I'm here to help. For now, just sit up, sit back and read on to see if this sounds like you.

Symptoms

- Tight, achey shoulders and neck, shoulder blades and areas surrounding the neck

- Dull soreness, sometimes sharp or stabbing pain between shoulder blade or in the actual shoulder joint

- Headaches, tingling and knotted up neck, jaw and shoulders

Treatment

I believe it was Sir Issac Newton that stated for every action there is an equal and opposite reaction. Hell, he made a friggin' law about it. So, in the world of exercise physics... when you start to experience tightness because of rounding of the spine, forward head tilt and rolling of the shoulders, the natural reaction would be to open up your chest and flex your spine and look towards the sky... the opposite motions to what got you there in the first place. I've included this sample shoulder and neck mobilizer exercise program and a stretch program to help aide in recovery and avoid at all costs the hunch back of Notre Dame vibe. *Check Appendix A.1 for descriptions of each exercise and A.2 for definitions of the exercise variables.*

SHOULDERS & NECK STRETCHES

Stretch (to be completed before every workout and as desired for up to 4 weeks)	Sets	Reps	Intensity	Tempo	Rest
A1. Pec Major/Minor Wall Stretch	1-2	2-3/side	BW	10/(10)	0
B1. Trap Lateral Stretch	1-2	2-3/side	BW	10/(10)	1min
C1. SB Lat Stretch	1-2	10	BW	10/(10)	30s
D1. Sub-Occipital Stretch	1-2	10	BW	10/(10)	30s

SHOULDERS & NECK EXERCISES

Exercise (to be completed every other day for up to 4 weeks)	Sets	Reps	Intensity	Tempo	Rest
A1. Shoulder Clocks	1-2	10/side	BW	breathing	10s
A2. Scap Pushups	1-2	10	BW	333	1min
B1. Wall Angels	1-3	10-15	BW	505	30s
B2. Face Pulls	1-3	10-15	BW	303	30s
B3. Neck Rolls	1-3	10-15	BW	breathing	1min
C1. Cat/Cow	1-2	10	BW	10/(10)	10s
C2. Quadruped Shoulder Twister	1-2	10/side	BW	333	30s

Elbows and Wrists

For every musician, the second area I see a whole bunch of nasty is in the elbow, forearm and in the wrists. This often stems from the problems in the shoulders (the whole upper extremity is connected, so oftentimes problems rooted in the shoulders and neck show themselves in the elbows or wrists and vice versa). However, a large part of a musicians' job requires them to hold their instrument with their hands clasped for minutes, if not hours at a time. Count the time of performance coupled with practice and depending on the individual this could be a majority of their time each and every friggin' day! To put it into perspective, think about making a fist and holding that fist for upwards of an hour. How's your hand feel after that? Pretty terrible, right? Imagine compounding that over the course of a few years, maybe 10, 20, 30? All that tightness creates a major imbalance in the forearm extensors and can lead to some much more serious problems. You've probably heard of carpel tunnel syndrome, tennis elbow and maybe even the term *tendonosis*. *A* lot of people mistakenly call this overuse syndrome "tendonitis". But actually, the *-itis* means resulting from an acute trauma, like you snap your wrist funny... not after repetitive movement like we tend to see in musicians. Well, these issues are common place for those that don't take the time to stretch and care for their body. Here are a few of the common symptoms, and the proper treatment.

Symptoms

- Sharp shooting pain on either side of the elbow, into the forearms and wrists

- Immobility and/or "clicking" in the wrist and/or elbow

- Tight forearms, dull/sore pain, fire or burning pain throughout forearm and wrists

Treatment

Again, the nature of the job as a guitar, strings, brass, or woodwind player demands holding on to the instrument for long periods of time. The same exercise physics hold true for the wrists and elbows as we focus on opening up the hands and stretching the wrists to increase range of motion on the meaty part under the forearm. The problem exists because of wrist and bicep "flexion" so we will look at stretching those muscles and "rebalancing the wheel" with corrective exercise. Here's a good stretch and exercise combo to help you combat the common problems of the wrist and elbows without causing further damage. *Check Appendix A.1 for descriptions of each exercise and A.2 for definitions of the exercise variables.*

ELBOWS & WRISTS STRETCHES

Stretch (to be completed before every workout and as desired for up to 4 weeks)	Sets	Reps	Intensity	Tempo	Rest
A1. Bicep Wall Stretch	1-2	2-3/ side	BW	10/(10)	0
A2. Tricep Wall Stretch	1-2	2-3/ side	BW	10/(10)	1min
B1. Forearm Extensor Stretch	1-2	3-5	BW	10/(10)	30s
B2. Forearm Flexor Stretch	1-2	3-5	BW	10/(10)	30s

ELBOWS & WRISTS EXERCISES

Exercise (to be completed every other day, alternating with shoulder/neck program for up to 4 weeks)	Sets	Reps	Intensity	Tempo	Rest
A1. Modified Reverse Grip Push Ups	2-3	10	BW	202	10s
A2. Bench Dips	2-3	10	BW	202	1min

Lower Back and Hips

Ahhh, the lower back. Undoubtedly one of the most common areas in our body to get injured, become sore and cause us great amounts of grief in our day-to-day lifestyle. So why does the back get so messed up? Most commonly the lack of strength and flexibility in the back leads to a strain when you lift improperly or twist suddenly. Again, improper movement. So you could imagine how vulnerable the back of a musician, roadie, engineer or stage tech would be. All of these professions have duties that compromise posture and some compound that by moving heavy things like amps and stage gear. Now, I've grouped the hips in here as well, and I'll tell you why. There's a group of muscles known in layman's terms as the "hip flexors" that play an integral part in lower back mobility. Now, without getting into too much of the exercise and kinesiology components of it all, part of this group of muscles loops in around your hip bone and ties-in up into your lower back. So, long story- short… if the hip flexors are messed up, there's a good chance your lower back will take on some of that noise. Some ways to alleviate the lower back pain and compression of the spine are simple strength exercises and gentle stretching or range of motion focused drills to increase flexibility through the affected areas to help release the tightness. Check it out below. I've listed common symptoms and then a proper treatment plan to help you keep that back of yours in top form.

Symptoms
- Dull, achey pain right atop the bum or hips. Generally central, however can be favoured to one side or the other

- Tight, stiff pain in the hip joints and/or lower back

- Poor range of motion and/or flexibility of hips and/or back

- Sharp, burning pain in front or side of hips and/or across lower back

Treatment

Well, for most musicians, just moving more with proper patterns without any serious resistance will make a huge difference in lower back and hip mobility. The trouble is when we sit (or stand) to practice, our bodies don't have the chance to move. This causes tightness and discomfort in the affected areas. The fix? Mobility drills to open up those areas and then strength drills to condition the body to endure the long hours of practice, loading gear or whatever the case may be. If you experience any sort of back pain, I'd like you to try the sample workout three times a week. Even if you don't feel any of the symptoms, you should be proactive and do these drills anyways. If you get an achey back, it can seriously reduce your drive to play and practice. *Check Appendix A.1 for descriptions of each exercise and A.2 for definitions of the exercise variables.*

LOW BACK & HIPS STRETCHES

Stretch (to be completed before every workout and as desired for up to 4 weeks)	Sets	Reps	Intensity	Tempo	Rest
A1. Supine (Single-leg) Glute Stretch	1-2	10/side	BW	10/(10)	0
B1. Windshield Wiper	1-2	2-3/side	BW	303	0
C1. McKenzie Press Up	1-2	10	BW	breathing	0
D1. "Wag the Tail"	1-2	10/side	BW	333	0
E1. Childs Pose	1-2	1	BW	1-2min hold	0

LOW BACK & HIPS EXERCISES

Exercise (to be completed every third day for up to 4 weeks)	Sets	Reps	Intensity	Tempo	Rest
A1. Supine Hip Raise	2-3	10-15	BW	202	15s
A2. SB Lower Body Rotation	2-3	10/side	SB	202	15s
A3. MB Russian Twist	2-3	10/side	8-10lbs	101	15s
A4. Supermans	2-3	10	BW	10/(5)	15s
A5. Waiters Bow	2-3	10	BW	555	2min

Chapter 3: What Every Musician Ever Needs To Know About Movement In Order To Prevent Having A Body That Always Hurts, All Of The Time

I have always maintained a strong relationship with the gym, fitness and training. But I'm a weird musician. I grew up playing sports at a competitive level, so exercise and activity and all that goes with it was second nature to me. It was a culture that was ingrained into my childhood, adolescence and early adulthood as a competitive speed skater. Not too many full-on musicians and industry folk have that same upbringing, so I can totally understand if this stuff seems way out there for you. Rest assured, beyond these pages we'll make sure you're comfortable incorporating the practice into your lifestyle in a way that you can dig. It's a lot different going out for a quick jog in the morning or hitting a weight session after lunch than it is sitting in rehearsal or in a studio session all day. But trust me, speaking from experience and from the number of people I have had in case study, the balance between proper movement and productivity, longevity in the game and overall wellbeing is paramount. You need to find it or you can bet your ass you won't last in the industry.

So let's talk about the key concepts of movement training that will prevent you from the aforementioned problems. I like to break it down into three simple bits, easy to remember and easy to incorporate (even if you're a drummer!).

1. Flexibility/mobility

2. Resistance/strength

3. Cardiovascular endurance

Unlike a lot of physical fitness literature out there in the testosterone-fuelled online world of bloggers and websites that promise you to "get ripped, fast!" or "get a 6 pack in 6 weeks", there is no best form of exercise. Fact is, all three of the above (strength, mobility and endurance) are key for you as a musician to live the best quality of life you can. You're kind of swimming upstream with regards to the lifestyle choices that are typically associated with this industry already. There's a lot of booze, a lot of poor eating, a lot of sleepless nights and so much party. All the party. Which is totally cool, I'm not going to judge, heck, I am a part of it. There are some people that get into this line of work explicitly for that kind of lifestyle. But don't be naive. It'll wear on you over time and your body can only physically take so much abuse. Stop reading and throw this book away or give it to your grandmother for her birthday or something if you're not down with this. This next bit is for the serious musicians that want to excel in performance, day in day out. No excuses. Let me show you how to *manage*, not remove, the lifestyle elements that hinder physical well-being with the above listed three fundamental concepts of movement training. First up, Flexibility and Mobility.

Flexibility & Mobility

99% of the new clientele (or "athletes" as I like to classify my clients) that I see have some sort of mobility issues or are just plain inflexible. This is so, so, so common because of our general sedentary lifestyle, regardless of occupation. We just don't move as much as we once did when it was quite literally survival of the fittest. Those who weren't as fast as the next dude in the neighbouring village didn't eat. Think back to the kids' books...

you didn't see a bunch of fat cavemen, did you? Nah, they were all Greek Gods, Herculean-esque manly-men. Except for Barney and Fred, but I digress… The association with caveman and exercise is still predominant in the fitness world today, we now call it "functional exercise" and things like "primal movements" are at the top of most (good) personal trainers', health coaches and other industry professionals' *To Do* list. (Don't worry…we'll break down the movements later in the following chapters) And for me, primal movements are the root of my training philosophy. That said, without a solid grasp of mobility and flexibility, you're not getting very far with those primal patterns. I'd encourage you to pick up a few mobility accessories so you can add them to your training duffle bag. We'll get to that in a bit, but first let's walk you through what I do with my clients when we are first starting out to help aide in their mobility and flexibility training.

Movement Prep & Warm-Ups For Every Musician Ever

I've seen a lot of… interesting… warm ups from gym enthusiasts over the years. Nothing really surprises me anymore. From dudes shadow-boxing in the mirrors and lifting up their shirts (to check their abs I would assume), to gals sitting on the yoga mats for the whole morning, cellphone in hand switching from downward dog to Instagram selfie pose. Perhaps they're tweeting it…? Who knows… It's incredible, really.

I'm going to give you my take on warming up. I believe the whole point of warm up is to not only physically get the body warm, but neurologically start to prime the whole session and get you psychologically ready for your training. That means connecting mind and body in a sense that when we ask the body to do a little bit more resistance, or maybe push a little bit further into that stretch, it doesn't crap out or get injured. Make sense?

I can't tell you how many times I've been witness to a trainer telling their client to go hit the treadmill for a 10 minute warm up jog because "we've got a big, heavy chest day today!". Like WTF does jogging have to do with your chest? Sure, you get some blood flow, but there's no priming of those muscles YOU'RE ASKING TO LIFT REALLY HEAVY OBJECTS UP AND PUT THEM BACK DOWN, is there? I can't stress how frustrating it is when maybe two days later that same client comes back in complaining about how sore their shoulders are or how they've got a pinch in the back or something... no kidding. Maybe a light jog will fix it up...? Eff'. My. Life. If you're going to focus on a specific area to gain strength, power, mobility, etc... focus a mobilizing and engaging preparation for that movement and that group of muscles. Period. End of story.

For me, movement prep is simple. I incorporate a practice of moving from the most supported (least likely to injure and very simple movements) to least supported (most challenging and more suspect to cause injury) in a progressive fashion. Basically, I take a client from lying down on their back to standing on their feet, without injury in a little over 10 minutes, maybe 20 if we're brand new. It looks a little something like this: *Check Appendix A.1 for descriptions of each exercise and A.2 for definitions of the exercise variables.*

MOVEMENT PREP & WARM-UP

Exercise (to be completed before every workout)	Sets	Reps	Inten sity	Tempo	Rest
A1. Supine Hip Raise	1-3	10-15	BW	Breathing	15s
A2. Supine Knee Drop	1-3	10/ side	BW	Breathing	15s
A3. "Shoulder Check" Cobra	1-3	10/ side	BW	Breathing	15s
A4. Horse Stance, Dynamic	1-3	10/ side	BW	Breathing	15s
A5. Stationary Lunge	1-3	10/ side	BW	Breathing	15s
A6. Inchworm	1-3	10	BW	Breathing	15s

Now, don't get hung up on the actual exercise. You can pretty much get away with (and I'd encourage you to do so) any type of bodyweight movement, stretch or strength that you like. Rather I'd like you to remember the format of supported to unsupported. From the top of your movement prep you'd perform a drill;

A1. From your back (or "supine")

A2. That incorporates rotation

A3. From face down (or "prone")

A4. From hands and knees (or "quadruped")

A5. From a kneeling stance (or "split stance")

A6. From your feet (either single foot or with both touching)

As you get more comfortable with this warm up concept, the total time that you take to complete it will lessen. You'll be more mobilized and well rehearsed in these movements so your body won't struggle with adapting to the priming of the associated muscles. Plus, you'll get to feel what areas of your body may need a bit more attention than the others, and if you know what the basis of your program is for that day (ie. big, heavy chest day) you'll be better prepared to prime that spot (ie. more focus on the upper body, shoulders/chest area) and not waste time on areas that aren't as crucial for that day (ie. 10 minute jogs before chest day...WTF?).

Accessory Equipment to Help Every Musician Ever With Piss-Poor Mobility

In the world of fitness, there's a lot to take in. In regards to mobility, there's even more. It's quickly become a real trend in the industry (thank God!) in supporting a healthy and active lifestyle. That said, I'll let you know what things you need and what things you don't really need to support maintaining the rock star lifestyle. Here it goes:

Musts vs. Busts: On The Road

Mobility & Flexibility "Musts" For Every Musician Ever	Why?	Mobility & Flexibility "Busts" For Every Musician Ever	Why?
Foam Travel Roller	Light, convenient way to alleviate tightness and muscle soreness	Wobble/ balance board	Functionality. Unless you're performing in the circus…rarely will you need to be on one foot, slaying a solo while juggling an infant from a slack line.
Lacrosse Ball	Great for "pinning" procedures in recovery	Stretching machines	Each individual has their own rage of motion that's natural. A machine is going to compromise that natural range.
Heavy Stretch Band	Great for myofascial stretching treatments	Aggressive therapy tools & equipment	Generally beyond the practical sense of what recovery is about
Yoga mat	Provides a clean, comfortable area to stretch on the road	Miracle pills that promote better mobility or flexibility	There are no shortcuts. Do the work. Stretch.

Part 2: Nutrition

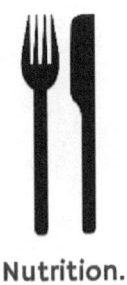

Nutrition.

"The food you eat can be either the safest and most powerful form of medicine or the slowest form of poison."

— *Ann Wigmore*

BETWEEN TWO AISLES: WITH KIRBY CRIDDLE

In the spring of 2016, en route to Canadian Music Week, we made a stop in Saskatoon. One of my dear friends (*singer-songwriter, yogi, Reiki Master, alternative health care pro, owner/operator of Illuminara Wellness and just generally badass, awesome human being and magnetic soul*) Kirby Criddle and I got together for the afternoon to hang out. Knowing what Kirby knows, I wanted to shamelessly exploit her knowledge and education in the world of nutrition. She also comes from two very polar-opposite backgrounds; Proactive Alternative Health and the Canadian indie roots music scene. We decided to go into Dad's Organic Market, a family owned and locally operated whole food grocer full of folks that seemed to be Kirby's nearest and dearest family. She has the warmest heart so it's easy to mistake complete strangers for lifelong friends around her. We cruised the aisles of Dad's for about an hour and filmed some great footage to help other musicians make more health conscious (and cost-effective) nutritional decisions while on the road. From bananas, to peanut butter, the difference between kefir and Greek yogurt to the benefits of Kombucha on the road.. we discussed it all. It's really amazing to experience a tour with healthy food options to choose from instead of making the Timmy's and McD's stops each day. You really feel the difference. Much more energy. If you're interested, message me. I'll email you links to the videos.

Please visit Dad's Organic Market if you find yourself in Regina or Saskatoon. They were great to us and the products they carry at an affordable price point are worth your visit alone. Treat yourself to the proper fuel.

Chapter 4: What Every Musician Ever Needs To Know About Nutrition In Order To Become A Road Warrior

There are three rules when it comes to surviving on the road:

1. Don't sacrifice nutrition for low cost, poor quality junk

2. Stay hydrated

3. Prepare meals and pack your snacks whenever possible

Let's dive in to these points...

Don't Sacrifice Your Nutrition. Period.

You will quickly realize that those extra few dollars up front to buy ice, a cooler and pack some celery, peanut butter and kefir would have been a better option over the 3 straight days of Wendy's and Tim Hortons on the Vancouver to Winnipeg stretch. Puke. Not only does fast food (I consider any food that's not raw, or natural, home grown, prepared by yourself or store bought without preservatives as "fast food") play with your energy levels and provide you with inadequate nutrition, but the crap you get in the chemicals is highly addictive and refined. This means your body goes through a roller coaster of emotional response after you down a bag of chips or a donut and double double and you're much more likely to continue this trend of binging because your system is craving nutrients and sending out triggers to get you to the nearest gas station to fulfill those requests. It's insane. It's also a black hole. You crave more artificial food (or more accurately, the chemicals in the said artificial food) the more artificial food you eat! Bahhh! And down that rabbit hole you go. How cool would it be if you just ate a low glycemic real piece of fruit (I'll explain the glycemic index in the next few pages) with some organic peanut butter and as a result satisfied your cravings in one shot? With that, you've got a pretty good macro nutrient spread (again, I'll explain this in detail in a bit), and most importantly you'll tend to sustain energy hours after eating, something those Timmie's DD don't provide. Here's a good few steps in order to help you choose more nutritionally dense foods while on the road.

Choose Lower Glycemic Foods More Often

Low Glycemic Indexed foods (GI) is science code for foods that don't make you crazy energetic for an hour and then leave you wiped until your next spike. This blood sugar roller coaster effect plays a pivotal role in energy levels throughout the day, so when you're on a rollercoaster, your body isn't in as good shape because it's fighting to maintain a sense of normalcy.

Your nutrition can help or hinder this normalcy... so here are some great examples to help balance your blood sugar out through your fuel. Most proteins and healthy fats are great. Things like chicken, eggs, avocado, nuts and seeds, are great staples for your diet. Then as far as carbs go - cherries, apples, bananas, rice, sweet potatoes, carrots, all leafy greens... you know... the good healthy stuff you probably pass by en route to the Kraft Dinner or Uncle Ben's. Okay, maybe not. That was a sharp generalization and probably unfair, but it's kind of funny how we perceive value. Typically, we are more inclined to shop for the dollar/box of KD rather than grabbing a bunch of spinach, even though the nutritional value doesn't even compare and it might only be a few cents more than the Big Mac... I've said it before and I'll say it again, it just comes down to bringing about some nutritional awareness.

For a quick whirlwind of *what not to eat*, stay away any foods high in fructose, sucralose, glucose or any of the "ose's" as they're synonymous with "sugar high"… and also generally steer clear of foods that have a bunch of words you can't pronounce on the label. They'll also tend to make you spike and crash. You know, chocolate bars, candies and of course everyone's favourite - coffee and creamers.

So take a peek and see what areas you might be able to improve on if you tend to have crashes. Since I have found it more common that grains, cereals and other starch based carbohydrates find themselves in a typical musician's diet, I have listed a "this over that" styled comparison chart for you to make the right call on the road.

GLYCEMIC INDEX CARBOHYDRATE BASED FOODS (CANADIAN DIABETES ASSOCIATION)

Top Five High Glycemic Foods To Avoid	Top Five Low Glycemic Foods To Eat
French fries	Sweet potato/yams
Bagel	Pumpernickel bread
Pretzels	Pasta/Noodles
Soda Crackers	Chickpeas/Lentils
Corn Flakes/Rice Krispies	All Bran/Oat Bran

Stay Hydrated.

It'll help you avoid death or death-like symptoms. Seriously. I can't tell you how many times I have read (especially in the summer) some sort of headline that's like "Stage Manager On Big Festival Tour Collapses." Paramedics on site, all good in the hood. Buddy just needed to drink some water. Like really? It's one of the first things we learn as infants, but we now have to be reminded about drinking water? I'm going to give you three (that's right, only three) reasons your body (and that of every musician) needs to have ample amounts of water to aid in performance. Here they are:

1. Water improves cognitive function (that's the ability to think clearly…)

2. Water helps to avoid muscle cramping (that's the ability to move properly)

3. Water keeps you far away from exhaustion, coma and death (that's the ability to live properly)

Pretty self explanatory, right? Right. We need to be more diligent about this, folks. Too many music biz pros are collapsing on stage, experiencing physical deficiencies and worse yet, jeopardizing their health. Drink water.

Eat well, man.

When I hit the road nowadays, it's very rare that I don't pack at least a small cooler with some fresh produce, trail mix or raw nut bars and of course peanut or almond butter; a staple on the road (we'll get into that a bit later). When space isn't as limited I take a bigger cooler and ensure that the groups I am working with have a steady supply of whole foods, packed with nutrition at their disposal while logging the kilometres across the nation. It's so, so, so easy to pack a few key items! It takes just as long to do that in a town as it does to stop at the Timmies, or McD's on the way out. And OHMYGAWD, what a difference THAT makes.

I figured the most applicable way to communicate healthy eating habits on the road is by making super relevant, generalized conclusions drawn from what I've seen in my nearly ten years in the health industry, and then offering simple ways to remedy them. Again, I've narrowed it down to the Top 3 issues I see related to nutrition in the folks I work with. They are in no particular order, just what comes to mind:

1. Lack of energy and motivation
2. Soreness and stiffness
3. Always hungry/Lack of appetite

So you're lacking energy, eh?

Makes sense. Especially if you're living the typical gruelling road lifestyle of late nights, loads of booze and party and then off to the next town, 300km away...

I'm here to suggest that your food, or "fuel" might be hindering your performance as an artist and function as a human. Let's take a look at why.

Let's think of your body as a car. You have an exterior (generally hardened and weathered after a decade in this industry), and an interior (full of parts that are supposed to work as efficiently as possible when maintained properly). I want you to think of the exterior and the interior parts as unchangeable. You're not going to change them too much without serious work. Then you have outside elements like fluid levels, fuel and oil. I want you to think of these additional things as variables that may affect the performance of you, the car. Now, let's just say you're a sports car, because that's a high performing machine. You want to go fast, create excitement and win over the fans. 0-60 as fast as you can, looking great and repeating championships as many years down the road as possible.

Well, if you don't put oil in your car, or you throw sludge in to your gas tank and forget to top up the fluids, you can expect to run into problems, right? So why is nutrition such a hard concept to get behind? Expect shitty performance (ie. lack of energy and motivation) when you mix poor quality foods, not enough water and no additional supplements (vitamins and minerals) with a high demand, high stress lifestyle.

Rest assured, if this sounds like you then I have a simple fix. You'll need to commit though, can you do that?

Next time you're on the road, keep mindful as to when you're eating. One of the simplest ways to sustain energy throughout the day is by eating every few hours. Don't let your body get to the point of hunger or in most cases "hanger". Every 4 hours grab an apple, maybe some celery with peanut butter or a nice sit down with your band over a coffee and a hearty breakfast of toast, eggs and avocado. If you plan on eating nutrient dense, whole foods every few hours, you will not experience the highs and lows typically associated with processed fast food options on the road. Thus, you're much more likely to sustain energy and feel a bit more motivated!

So you're sore, stiff and achey all over, eh?

Pretty common theme amongst this crowd. I oftentimes start a conversation with a prospective new client with something like "Do you experience any aches or pains that never seem to go away?" 99% of the time I get a very decisive "yes!"

Most of us aren't well hydrated enough to actually know what it feels like to be, as I classify, "un-sore" (and yes, that's a scientific definition…) and therefore that feeling of chronic stiffness, sore achey muscles and poor flexibility is just a "normal" part of day-to-day living.

Newsflash! What our medical world labels "normal" and what is actually *healthy* are two VERY, very different things. For example, if you walk into a Safeway or a London Drugs to sit in the blood pressure cuff chair over in the pharmacy, "normal" blood pressure readings are listed as anything under 130/85 for the general population. This is total bullshit, seeing as though no more than 5 years ago we were all terrified if our blood pressure read higher than 120/80! (which is a more accurate definition of cardiac health if you ask me… but I digress…) So what lead to the change in what's *normal*, and why the eff are we suddenly okay with our baseline measurements creeping up the charts like any Drake track in 2015?

It doesn't take a medical bioengineer to conclude that the standard North American lifestyle plays a large role in what we deem as "normal" health nowadays. Denton et al conclude that the increase in certain dietary components (such as salt in the North American diet) increases hypertension. It makes sense. We eat a lot of processed foods. Processed foods have a ton of sodium to maintain shelf life. Eat more crap like that and your blood pressure will slowly rise. I will further suggest that increased work hours, sleep deprivation and general inactivity amongst a majority of the public plays a pivotal role in determining what is "normal". End of the day, what's *normal* and what's *healthy* are two different things. I don't have a scholarly article to support that, but I think that is just common sense.

So how do we get out of this sore, stiff, achey rut? Because that's not healthy, even though you may think it's normal. So, let's talk about getting healthy!

ANTI-INFLAMMATORY VS. INFLAMMATORY FOODS

"We shouldn't put age limits on our dreams. Most of us do not have thousands of dollars to spend on our health and bodies. Diet is the simplest and most clear cut method to continue our passion and pursue our dreams late into life." - Dara Torres, Olympic Silver Medalist

Inflammation occurs in many forms and is actually a part of a healthy immune system as according to Rosen & Witinok-Huber (Anti-Inflammatory Foods). Discolouration, tightness, inflexibility, pain, swelling… these are all symptoms of inflammation. Fortunately, as the leading quote to start this chapter suggests, our diet plays a huge role in keeping this stuff minimal. So let's talk about anti-inflammatory foods. These are foods high in nutrients that tend to keep the effects of inflammation in, on, or around our bodies low.

Here's a list of my favourite real, raw, whole foods that'll help keep that soreness at bay:

Anti-Inflammatory Foods (Eat lots of these!)

- Nuts
- Fish (wild salmon especially) and Omega 3 fatty foods or fish oil capsules* *in place of fish… as toxins in farmed fish are still prevalent, ie. mercury levels are still wicked high*
- Spices like turmeric, ginger and garlic
- Leafy greens like spinach and kale
- Fruits, most notably berries

- Sweet potatoes

Surely there's something on this list that you can be eating more of, right? Okay, that's a start. I find it easier to coach the folks I'm working with into adding something, rather than removing things from their current lifestyle. It just works out better and is generally more positive. However, I feel it's important for everyone to know the things that aren't helping contribute to a healthy lifestyle. That said, here are a few foods that make for a more irritable digestive system:

Inflammatory Foods (Cut back on these!)

- Processed sugars (…are everywhere.. if you don't believe me, stay tuned for the next chapter)
- Refined carbohydrates (anything boxed in aisle 22… you know, right beside the box of Oreo's)
- Dairy; milk, cheese, ice cream (we don't need these in our diet at all)
- Hydrogenated Oils (bad, bad, bad for the heart…)
- Beef, pork (red meats in general are hard to break down and hard for the body to process)

Now, remember. I'm not preaching a certain dietary path when I suggest these principles. It's just food for thought. However, if you tend to see issues like sore joints, trouble digesting certain foods and a weird kink in the neck, I AM suggesting that your diet may be the culprit. Take a look at what you're currently doing and go from there. I tend to follow a plant based diet, but still enjoy meats and animal byproducts like organic dairy and eggs, but that's just how my body responds best. You may be different and I'd encourage you to play around with things until you find a combination that works. You'll know when it does because those aches and pains that once were "normal", magically disappear over time. Amazing, really.

So you say you're always/never hungry, eh?

Hmm. This one's a kicker. In keeping with the theme, the food we eat is our fuel. Backtrack for a sec, the fuel in the gas tank of our car will last longer if it's higher quality, right? When dealing with humans, the same thing applies. So let's start with addressing those of you that have the "I eat and eat and eat all day and never seem to be full" dilemma.

Always Hungry

Problem:

Aside from the small chance that you could be missing an enzyme or have a medical condition (in which I strongly advise you to go see your trusted medical professional...) let's just cut the bullshit. You're not eating quality food. Even if your portions are small, quality foods will control that appetite at least a little bit. So, stop eating garbage because the garbage is ruining your guts, so that when you do finally have a good nutritious meal, your body can't even absorb the wholesome nutrients you're trying to fuel it with. It's a vicious circle!

Secondly, you're not drinking enough water. Oftentimes, our body tricks our mind into sending appetite signals to get some form of hydration because you're so friggin' pre-occupied with sending that Tweet or something that you forgot to eat/drink/piss in order to take basic care of yourself. Body goes, "Hey, buddy! Pay attention!" and sends the signal for a hunger (or "Hanger" at this point...) strike to get you off your butt and to the kitchen or more likely the nearest drive-thru, if you're on the road. Again, not the right approach.

Solution:

Eat higher quality foods, rich in anti-inflammatory nutrients (see list back a few pages) more often. Make sure you're eating something when you first get up. Here's why:

You're likely sleeping 4-6 hours. Unless you're a great multi-tasker and part circus freak, you're likely not eating whilst fast asleep, right? So, your body has been starved of nutrients (and hydration) for those 4-6 hours already. **WHY ON EARTH WOULD YOU CONTINUE TO STARVE IT FOR ANOTHER FEW HOURS?** It's really silly to (particularly when you read that out loud), but we do it. I can't even tell you how many people I first start working with that aren't eating something upon waking. Yet these same people complain about being hungry throughout the day. Well, set the intention when your day begins. Eat something. Get the body some nourishment ASAP. You'll start the process right off the hop and things will be better throughout the day. Promise.

As for the water thing. The solution to not drinking enough water is, and I know… this might be surprising… but **DRINK MORE WATER.** End of story. I don't care how. For those of you that don't like the "taste" of water, if that is indeed a thing, flavour it with lemon or lime or cucumber. Yep, slice that stuff up and plunk it in and slam a few water bottles each day. Here's a good way to know you're having enough water throughout the day.

1. Take your favourite water bottle (750ML -1L) and fill it with water (and lemon/lime/cucumber if desired)

2. Grab 4 hair elastics or rubber bands and put them on said water bottle.

3. Take a rubber band off of the bottle every time you fill up. That way, you know you've had at least 3 litres of water each day, which is a good start for the typical human.

Never Hungry

Problem:

This one's a little harder to assess, and may need help from a medical professional. You may not feel hungry because your energy requirements for the day have been met. However, in rare circumstances it could be a sign of something bigger, such as kidney disease or cancer so it's always good to speak to a doctor. The biggest thing is knowing the difference between not actually being hungry and not *wanting* to eat. The latter could be a sign of a psychological issue such as anorexia and I would strongly advise speaking with your trusted medical professional if this sounds like you.

Solution:

It's out of my scope of practice to recommend anything for further medical issues so I will leave it up to you after you talk to a medical professional. I will say that from a physiological standpoint, our appetite is driven by our energy and nutrient demands. So if you're not hungry, like ever… there's a good chance that you're not moving, like ever…

Does this sound like you?

Fix that. Start moving a bit each day. Nothing crazy. Just get up and go for a walk in the morning before you start your day. Or join a friend at the gym or do a drop-in class at the yoga studio down the block. Find a way to burn some daily calories and you may start to see an increase in your appetite.

Chapter 5: What Every Musician Ever Needs To Know About Food Labels

HIP HOP SAVED ME...

You know, I'm totally not embarrassed to admit I had no idea what those numbers on the side of a can or boxed meal meant. I was even two years into my career in the fitness industry! No idea! So I can only imagine what someone that focuses on what scales to play and what key to sing in or what strings to buy for their Fender is going through when they hit aisle nine in Safeway...

It took me moving out on my own and living in Kelowna, British Columbia while going to UBCO in the Cultural Studies Program to really understand how to go about preparing food. I learned this from LL Cool J. So yes, hip hop saved me. He and his trainer Dave Honig teamed up with Jeff O'Connell to put out an exercise & nutrition book focused on smart and simple ways to live a healthier lifestyle and look good naked. Let's be honest, that's 99% of the population's number one reason we subject ourselves to the hardships of exercise. I have no problem admitting that. However, I learned a lot of stuff about the smallest changes that make the biggest difference and I want to pass along something I think us musicians will find invaluable while travelling on the road and considering our nutrition and lifestyle choices.

Again, I'm not trying to remove the party from the lifestyle, I'm just going to suggest some things that you can choose to implement or not. If it works for you, my job is done. To start, let's look at food labels. If you're going to eat food, you should probably know what it is you're actually eating, right?

How To Read A Food Label

As LL and Honig suggest in the *Platinum Workout,* those percentages you see on the side of a food label DO mean something. I have included two Canadian food labels for us to take a look at. My apologies for the shitty quality of images, I'm a starving artist/author, so I'm still waiting on the royalty cheques. Until they come in, you'll have to deal with these blurred images.

Example A.   Example B.

Nutrition Facts	
Serving Size 1 bar (2 lbs)	
Servings Per Package 1	
Amount	% Daily Value
Calories 4600	
Fat 260 g	400 %
Saturated 160 g	800 %
+ Trans 0 g	
Cholesterol 200 mg	120 %
Sodium 1400 mg	40 %
Carbohydrate 960 g	320 %
Dietary Fiber 40 g	
Sugars 840 g	
Protein 120 g	
Vitamin A 0 % Vitamin C 0 %	
Calcium 320 % Iron 80 %	

Nutrition Facts / Valeur nutritive	
Serving 3" X 4" piece (214 g)	
pour morceau de 3" x 4" (214 g)	
Amount / Teneur	% Daily Value / % valeur quotidienne
Calories / Calories 280	
Fat / Lipides 11 g	17 %
Saturated / saturés 1 g	5 %
+ Trans / trans 0 g	
Cholesterol / Cholestérol 35 mg	
Sodium / Sodium 110 mg	5 %
Carbohydrate / Glucides 46 g	15 %
Fibre / Fibres 4 g	16 %
Sugars / Sucres 32 g	
Protein / Protéines 3 g	
Vitamin A / Vitamine A	2 %
Vitamin C / Vitamine C	15 %
Calcium / Calcium	2 %
Iron / Fer	8 %

As you can see (hopefully), at first glance it may be hard to pick out the little things on these labels that may influence your purchasing decision. Listed below is a step-by-step of how to analyze these two. There are certain things that are mandatory on a Canadian Food label, and other things that are optional. I'll dissect the above examples for you and you can have a closer look next time you're in aisle nine, choosing between six boxes of Kraft Dinner or four cans of tuna.

Serving Size

Pretty self explanatory, but when you think about comparing two foods, if one is measured in 2 lbs and the other is in 214g there's a significant difference and that will skew the percentages that follow if you're not mindful of that. That said, you'll tend to pick up the item that has the smaller amount of calories, sugars, sodium etc… thinking you're making a smart choice, when really, the company knew that and adjusted their serving size accordingly. It's pretty sneaky, right?

% Of Daily Value (% DV)

This number tells us if the serving has a little or a lot of the nutrient in it. 5% is a little and over 15% is a lot. How % DV is calculated is by dividing the amount of the serving size of a nutrient by the daily total amount then multiplying it by 100 (to find the daily values of nutrients, please head to www.healthycanadians.gc.ca)

Calories

Also, pretty self-explanatory. This is the caloric amount per serving size. Calories, for those that aren't familiar, are basically the way we measure energy when dealing with nutrition. More calories = more energy! This is important for deciding how much food we need to eat, as input does equal output, those of us that move more and are larger in size require more calories per day. Makes sense, right? Keep that in mind when you're wondering why the waistline continues to grow (or shrink). We won't get into much more about the types of calories in this book, but know that different types of foods have higher caloric counts than others.

Fat

You guessed it. This is the amount of fat that's in the portion size, broken down into saturated and trans for your convenience. What's saturated fat you ask? Saturated fat, is an unprocessed fat found in our natural environment. For years, saturated fat has been labelled as an unhealthy fat, but this is likely due to just misinformation and the pressure from big corporations trying to sell their products that were created without saturated fats. Humans have evolved gathering coconuts and hunting and using all parts of animals for years. Animal fats and tropical oils (palm, coconut and cacao) contain high amounts of saturated fats, so I am confused as to why we still have this unfounded fear of saturated fat.

Trans fat, on the other hand is an "unhealthy" fat. They've had an additive to prolong their life, actually making them non-perishable in most cases. Products such as margarine and most shelf stable cooking oils (safflower, soybean, corn oil) are notorious for having high trans fat content and can severely alter your health and performance. Avoid these guys. It's like eating plastic.

Cholesterol

Much like with saturated fat, the medical world has made cholesterol out to be the bad guy. However, cholesterol is a naturally produced molecule in the body that helps with tissue and membrane repair. The body produces more when we don't eat foods high in cholesterol. With that said, if I don't eat enough, my body will trigger production of more. Cholesterol doesn't have to be bad, but the key here is the transport, HDL or LDL. Without getting into it too deep, just know that HDL is the good stuff that you want in your diet to help mop-up excess cholesterol and bring it to the liver. Your best bet is just to go get your blood cholesterol tested and ensure it's under 150mg/dl to avoid heart disease problems in the future. Studies show that there are virtually zero cases of heart disease or cardiovascular problems in people with cholesterol levels lower than 150mg/dl.

Sodium

Sodium (not to be confused with salt, which contains sodium), is an essential mineral,. That means your body doesn't produce it naturally, therefore, you must obtain it through food. As Precision Nutrition explains, sodium is key in absorption of glucose, water, chloride and amino acids, and helps to maintain electrochemical gradient across cell membranes (which means the body can send and receive electrical signals) which helps muscle contraction, nerve impulse transmission and cardiac function. If you don't have enough sodium you may experience nausea, vomiting, cramps, fatigue and disorientation. However, too much sodium results in diarrhea, abdominal cramps, vomiting and nausea among other symptoms. Some foods that are rich in sodium are: whole grains, whole fruits, vegetables, lean meats and legumes. So basically just eat a balanced diet and you shouldn't hit either extreme.

Carbohydrate

Yeah, there's a lot of misinformation out there on carbs. People tend to think only grains and starch based foods count as carbs and think that they're eating carb-free if they avoid pastas and breads and the like. But then I ask, "Okay so no fruits, or vegetables or sugars in your diet?"

"Of course I eat those!" Well, then you eat carbs. On a food label, carbs are broken down into dietary fibre and sugars. You want to have a higher portion of fibre and a lower portion of sugars for the total carbohydrate content of the serving.

Protein

Protein is a macronutrient that is essential in rebuilding cell tissue and proper day-to-day functioning. Without it, your body doesn't work right. It also helps to regulate body fat (as according to Precision Nutrition) through the production of glucagon. What's glucagon? Glucagon helps to signal the liver to break down glucose. So how much protein do you need? Depends. That's why there's no percentage listed generally. The activity level of the individual is one determining factor. So in general it's good to pay attention to how much protein you are having in relation to how much moving you are doing, as extra will be converted slowly into sugars.

Vitamins, Calcium & the rest of the label

The last little bit on a food label contains things such as vitamins and calcium; important nutrients and minerals that aide in the regular function of the body. Nothing too crazy here, just figure out if you're getting enough of your vitamins by actually reading these values. Recovery from deficiencies can be a long road, so talk to your trusted health professional if you have any questions about where you may be lacking in these departments.

Chapter 6: Three Simple Recipes For Every Musician Ever

Typically, there are three meals per day; breakfast, lunch and dinner. I'm going to give you one really simple meal I've crafted up for each meal time so you limit your excuses as to why you can't eat healthy. First up -

Breaky:

Peanut Butter & Banana Protein Shake

Ingredients

- 250ml almond milk/water

- 1 large banana

- 1 tbsp organic peanut butter

- 1 scoop of vanilla Vega One protein powder

Optional

- 1 tsp of cinnamon

- 100ml of coffee

Instructions

Throw everything in a blender and turn the blender on. Boom. There you go. This is a quick way to get all the major macros, protein, carb and healthy fats in, first thing. Start your day right with this one!

Lunch:

Tuna, Veggie Rice Bowl

Ingredients

- 1 can of tuna
- 2 cups of frozen (or fresh preferably) veggies
- 1 cup of cooked long grain brown rice
- splash of apple cider vinegar

Optional

- Hot sauce

Instructions

Dump a bunch of water in a pot, splash your apple cider vinegar in with the mix and throw a cup of long grain brown rice in to soak for a minimum of 4 hours (best to leave it over night). Then strain the rice, add the correct portion of water and cook. By soaking the rice in apple cider vinegar you remove the natural defence mechanism of the grain and increase the digestibility. So it'll be better for you!

Once you cook the rice, half the battle is over. Now you should steam or pan fry your veggies up and once they're cooked, dump them into the rice. Crack open the can of tuna, dump it into the mix and presto! You've got a smorgasbord of health! Splash some hot sauce in there for flavour if you want, and go to town on a delicious lunch.

Dinner:

Chicken Spinach Salad

- 1 tbsp olive oil
- 2 tbsp apple cider vinegar
- 1 tbsp of sunflower seeds or unsalted, un-candied trail mix
- 1 chicken breast or 1 thigh (3oz)
- 2 cups of spinach

Instruction

Gently toss the spinach in a bowl with seeds, oil and vinegar. Then pan fry or roast your chicken and cut it up into bite size portions. Or don't. It's not my salad. Toss it all up in the bowl and voila! She's ready to go! A nice light dinner with a ton of good things going on. Get on it.

Part 3: Mindset

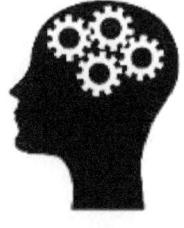

Mindset.

"You should sit in meditation for twenty minutes every day — unless you're too busy. Then you should sit for an hour."

— Zen proverb

OWNERSHIP, POSITIVITY & DOING THINGS FOR A GREATER GOOD

If I have learned anything over the course of the past few years or so, it's been that respect is earned and one's ability to command that respect comes back to how he or she handles situations that aren't "optimal" at best. For example, if you are going to make excuses about why you may or may not have missed a few notes on stage, be prepared to be confronted on it. If you can own it, cool. If those excuses start to deflect the fact that you screwed up, you're not getting much sympathy or - more importantly - respect from the likes of me… or agents, managers, A/R etc… just own it, okay? This is the first lesson I'm including in this the last part of this guide. I feel that this part of the reading is where it might get a little weird for the folks that might not have much familiarity with things like positive attitude, meditation and other stress management techniques… but I'm set on overcoming this along with a few other ways to incorporate a healthy mindset into your health and ultimately your performance both on and off stage. Buckle up, ladies and gentlemen. It's go time.

Chapter 7: Two Key Ingredients Every Musician Ever Needs To Have In Order To Become A Better Human

BE MINDFUL

Call it what you want. Mindfulness, consideration, thoughtfulness. Just put yourself in the other's shoes. Once you start to do as you want others to do unto you, you'll start being a better human. Period.

I find that once someone starts being an outstanding person, stress magically disappears from their lives, they take a more positive approach to handling tough situations and their actions are just a lot more professional in general. Strange, right? Be mindful and considerate and good things happen.

OWN YOUR SHIT

Nothing screams immaturity, unprofessionalism and disrespect more than some whiney rock star shouting at the sound guy/girl about not hearing themselves in a monitor, not having the right tone or something equally as ridiculous. How about you just play better? However, recognize the good stuff too. If you're doing something awesome, don't be afraid of acknowledging it. That said, if you 'eff' up, fess up to it. Simple as that. You're going to keep a lot more people around and maintain a certain level of respect if you can own your shit.

Some of you might be wondering what this has to do with mindset. Well, I'm a firm believer in respect for oneself as well as those around you. If you're lacking in either, it shows me that you either don't respect yourself, those around you or quite possibly both. That said, it's hard to carry forward a mindset strong enough to battle the road, deal with the highly stressful lifestyle of rock stardom and put up with all the political bullshit of the industry if you don't respect yourself or those around you, wouldn't you say? Imagine having the confidence to call the promoter, owning the fact that you might be later to the gig because you slept in. Not that the van had engine issues and your guitarist forgot his shoes so you had to turn around....blah blah blah.. how many people do you know that sound like this? Just full of excuses. I can tell you right now, important people stop paying attention to these folks sooner or later. Don't be one. That's why ownership is important. Cool? Cool.

I'm Trying To Hear Your Words, But Your Actions Are Just So Deafening...

I'd like to share a quick hypothetical story about ownership to really stress its importance. Let's say there was this bass player, lets call him Tim. Tim played in a group where I imagine much like many of you, Tim had a different vision of what success was. However, it took Tim a very long time to recognize this. Tim pushed the envelope on things that would further the band; making industry contacts, branching out and taking in events, hanging out after shows to mingle and getting out to other bands' shows around town to again reinforce their presence in the local scene. The rest of the band said they were on board with all of this. However, Tim rarely saw the action follow all the talk.

Tim wouldn't ordinarily have a problem with this. But it became frustrating to Tim when he would go ahead and do something that'd be ordinarily recognized as a good move (like book a tour) only to be met by resistance and a million excuses as to why the band shouldn't do that particular thing. At the end of the day, it just became clear that the priorities were different and the band didn't share the same vision of success as Tim. Not right. Not wrong. Just different and not something Tim wanted to be a part of.

How could this situation have been remedied? Well, honestly, Tim shouldn't care too much about how the rest of the group's interests didn't align with his. He *should* care that they *said* they were on board, but never followed through with the things that would have *shown* Tim that they were indeed in. All in. It's about ownership. If you can't follow through and own it, don't bother saying you will.

Chapter 8: Stress Relief 101 For Every Musician Ever -

Breathe, Smile, Sweat, Sleep

LIKE WHAT YOU DO, DO WHAT YOU LIKE.
Have you ever caught yourself doing something that you don't enjoy? Have you ever stopped and asked yourself why the eff you're doing it? This founding principle of what Simon Sinek classifies as "Finding Your Why" is something that a lot of people don't really consider until it's unfortunately much too late. My experience shows that breathing, smiling, sweating and sleeping promotes maximum productivity, a healthy lifestyle and ultimately the ability to recognize this "why". All it takes is the most basic of human functions connecting mind with body. Let's take a look.

BREATHE WITH ME...
Just as Prodigy suggests in the 1997 smash-hit "Breathe", breathing is important. Let's say our overarching goal is to achieve some sort of higher level of awareness. A higher level of consciousness. Let's just pretend that's the dream for a moment. Well, let's consider what all of these ancient practices like meditation and yoga and even the energizer series that I teach promote... breathing. Deep, conscious breathing. Why? Breath will calm the mind, releasing the chaos and disorganized energy from the mind down into the body to, in essence, promote a wicked abundance of energy your body can now use and deplete (you'll read how the mind and body coincide later in this

chapter…). If you don't believe me about how powerful your breath can be, try lying down before bed tonight, take a deep breath in for 7 seconds, then hold your breath for 7 seconds and then exhale for 7 seconds. Try to repeat this 7 times over but don't be shocked when you fall into a blissful snooze after the first few.

You should loosen up, feel your face soften, neck and shoulders drop and in general, feel more at ease. This is the first step. Keep mindful about how you feel and you will start to notice when you need to breath a bit more.

SMILE.

Be happy, man.

Next up - smiling. By smiling I really mean just be happy. There's not a lot in the world that should upset you to the point of ruining your day and I'd certainly argue there's a ton of stuff that can brighten your day if you look at it through a different lens.

> *"We are 100% able to change the outcome of any situation simply by how we react." - Mike Schwartz*

If you're having a hard time believing this statement, put it into practice. Here's a lofty example:

A singer steps up to the mic. Song opens up and singer forgets the lyrics. Singer now has a few options - Option A: Run off stage in a manic flee, Option B: make something up to cover the forgotten lyrics, or Option C: she lets the band repeat the intro and regains composure to sing the proper lyrics, just with a "live" performance kinda vibe a few bars late. Neither of these options are wrong, per se. But how the singer reacts ultimately changes what happens and the experience for everyone involved, right?

Depending on the lens you're looking through, the situations you're faced with may seem rather daunting. That's okay! I challenge you to take a step back on the next experience that you feel overwhelmed with and just breathe, smile and know that you have options.

Almost everything you do in life is a choice.

I say almost because there are some exceptions I'm sure. I personally haven't come across any that come to mind, but I'm only subject to my experiences. And in my experience, everything I've ever done is a choice. A *want* rather than a *need*. I've grown tired of hearing people say they "need to be somewhere in an hour", or they "need to go to work" or they don't "need to work out" etc…

No, of course not. You don't *need* to do any of that. You choose whether or not you carry out tasks such as going out, going to work or working out. You make the decision to fit those things in (or not) to your day. Don't try to blur a decision to do something with the feeling of necessity. You are not going to die because you *had* to eat that pizza. It's okay. Own it and move on. You wanted to eat that pizza. That salty, cheese-filled, tasty slice of heaven… Everything is a choice. Choose to remember that.

SWEAT.

"The body wants to move. Let it. The mind will follow."

Part of the smiling thing transpires from sweat (and movement). I've seen this first hand in working with what were once grumpy-ass human beings. These folks would come into my sessions, just poo-pooing the whole world around them. Sure enough by the end of our 60 minutes we had them chatting about their weekend and how they were looking forward to hanging out with their dog, nephews or whatever it may be. Totally different humans. What happened? Was this really all because they moved a little bit? Well, yes. Here's the science behind it.

Sweat is triggered when you start heating up and your body needs to cool down. Proper exercise triggers this response automatically as a defence mechanism so your body doesn't implode or anything crazy. When we exercise to a level that starts to produce sweat, we also trigger some good ol' hormones in the brain to be released. These endorphins or "happy" hormones trigger a feeling of euphoria and are common after completing a run (or similar task) at a level of intensity and/or volume that puts your body in a state of adaptation. Energy systems engage, blood starts pumping faster, lungs have to work harder to maintain oxygen flow to keep all systems go… these are all great things. And they're things that make the happy emotions come alive. The more you do it, the more noticeable it is to you (and others around you!) so keep it up. My general rule of thumb is to sweat once daily. I actually saw that quote on a Lululemon water bottle I once owned and I guess it just stuck. For some creative ideas to boost the sweat factor in your life, refer to all the stretch and workouts programs in Part 1 of this book.

SLEEP.

The body requires full attention all day and all night. To ensure this, you must sleep your eight hours or you will not be the very best version of yourself and that is the crime of the century.

I still love getting asked about how I wake up each morning, same time, regardless if I have clients that morning or not. Sometimes I'm out way past my bedtime too, and without fail I'm up by 6:30. Well, it's something I've had to work at, that's for sure. In the old days I would have slept until my body wanted to wake up, which sometimes when I was getting in from gigs at three or four am, meant the whole following day was shot. Waking up at noon was no longer cool. I needed to get things done. So I did a little research...

The Circadian Rhythm: "Almost all owls are nocturnal. So therefore most owls are night owls. Just sayin'..."

This next bit is all about how the sun and the moon and the winds operate, so if you're not into that kind of "airy-fairy hippy bullshit" you should skip ahead. However, if you give a damn about the way you feel, how long you live and actually making good use of your time on the planet, it might be worth the read.

The Circadian Rhythm, or "sun cycle" is the natural body clock that tells us humans when to wake up and get shit done. It's responsible for a lot of physiological responses in our bodies so it's pretty fundamental in helping us operate at our prime. This natural body clock is affected by many different factors, some internal such as stress hormones and some external such as sunlight and temperature. So, that said, if you screw up your sleeping schedule by playing shows early into the morning, you need to learn how to effectively manage that so you can still be optimal in performance night in, night out.

Here's a quick breakdown of your ideal 8 hours of sleep. And yes, it is important to sleep during these windows if you want to maximize your body's performance. You can't just make up the sleep by sleeping later in the day.

10pm - 2am Physical Repair

These are the hours that, with proper sleep (and quality production of growth hormones) your body will repair the cells that were destroyed through the course of the day. This is important in order to heal from physical injury as one can imagine, so if you're skipping out on these hours and you have a sore back, hip or shoulder… I'd say this probably has something to do with it.

2am - 6am Physiological Repair

The body tends to repair itself between these hours (as according to Leigh Brandon, CHEK Institute blog) and poor quality of sleep can lead to many health issues including lethargy, increased body fat, anxiety, increased chance of sickness, decreased libido, joint aches, cognitive problems, gut problems poor performance and many more dysfunctions. As you can see, sleep is so, so, so important!

I learned how to recover under short timelines with my time training for competitive speed skating. We did so much fricken volume I felt like a broken old man most days. I prayed for the cold tubs to recover and being able to feel my legs again. A day off from training was absolutely amazing. Rare, but amazing. In any case, I picked up a few tricks that I'd like to pass along to you to help you make the most of your situation.

"Three tricks of the trade to help recovery: Magnesium gel, Zinc and a good pillow"

Mike Schwartz

When I was speed skating, I learned very quickly how key recovery from physical stress was. Not only did the physical wear and tear knock me down, the mental game was incredibly draining. I found that my body and mind were both completely exhausted from the intensity of training sessions. In support of helping musicians see themselves as athletes, I believe that we need to treat the physical and psychological fatigue of a musician's lifestyle as we would a performance athlete.

So how do we do this? Well, aside from moving properly and eating the right foods, recovery is really dependent on well... recovering. That's right, sleep, rest and relaxation are all key factors in staying at your finest. That's cool, eh?

I have three tips that kind of blend the worlds of movement, nutrition and mindset for you. They've helped me recover, so start putting them into practice and see what happens.

1. Get into magnesium gel - Magnesium is second only to vitamin D in nutrient deficiency in the North American diet. We tend to eat a lot of processed foods and there's not a lot of room for essential minerals. Since our body doesn't produce magnesium on its own, we need to get it from outside sources. The gel (as opposed to magnesium citrate that you can buy in

pill form) provides a soothing effect and helps relieve muscle soreness. Applying this stuff on your legs and neck before bed will take down the effects of restless leg syndrome and let you sleep like a rock. Be sure to set a few alarms and start with a nickel sized amount in your hand. This stuff works like a dream. Seriously.

2. Load up on zinc - this natural aphrodisiac is one of 24 essential micronutrients that your body requires for proper function. It will help your recovery game by boosting testosterone and growth hormone, which aide in regeneration of cell tissue. Don't worry ladies, it won't boost your hormones too high, just enough so when you sleep you're actually repairing your body from the party the night before.

3. Get a good pillow. And use it - seriously. Go to a sleep specialist and figure out if you're a side, front or back sleeper and make an investment in yourself. This is such an important part of your wellbeing that if you maximize your rest, you'll perform better in all areas of life. That, I can promise. Also, when you're traveling on the road and sleeping in the van or hotel or wherever… that little piece of home will go a long, long way to keeping your body in the best alignment possible.

Chapter 9: Stress Relief 201 For Every Musician Ever -

Find Your Zen

After incorporating a mild dose of daily activity into your life and a bit more of a healthy attitude towards eating more nutrient dense foods, you may have a more positive outlook on life. You may start to notice things don't irritate you as much. Things just don't seem to upset you like they maybe would have 3 months ago. Yeah, since you've started doing a couple days of yoga each week, or even just stretching before you warm-up for rehearsal you've noticed a bit more energy and zest for life. Perfect.

This brings me to the last little bit of this part of the guide. Finding what it is exactly that gets you to that inner peace. In the holistic lifestyle coaching world, these are things known by us practitioners as "Peace Points". Let me elaborate:

A Peace Point is any activity that helps to distract us from the ordinary stresses of day to day life. A temporary vacation, if you will. These things can include but are not limited to: meditation, breathing drills, energizers (very popular in the CHEK Holistic Lifestyle Coach world. Contact me for more info on these types of drills), stretching, listening to relaxing music, writing, reading… etc. The purpose is the same; the activity doesn't matter. It brings us into a state of calmness, relaxation and cognitive (thinking) clarity. When you learn to incorporate something from the above list, you can control your reactionary responses much better. You are one with yourself and you are calm. Stress don't mean a thang! Seriously. It's empowering to realize this control. I like to call it self-realization of a zen state. I'd encourage you to find your zen and start incorporating just 5-10 minutes per day, sometimes more if you find yourself on the edge more often. It's seriously freeing.

Chapter 10: Stress Relief 301 For Every Musician Ever -

"Mind Sweat"

That's right. Mind sweat. It's an interesting theory I just came up with. Well, actually I probably didn't come up with the term. I'm sure I've heard it before. But here's what I mean by a sweating mind. The brain needs engagement. Just like any other organ, it can lose it's effectiveness if it's not being constantly utilized. Furthermore, when the brain is exposed to toxins, those toxins kill brain cells. That brain is now travelling upstream against the current. Over time, the decreased use of one's brain makes for a mind that isn't quite as quick, maybe has trouble recalling certain parts from past memories and starts to experience what is known as cognitive fogginess. That's right, just a little slower than the norm. Delayed reaction time, poor memory... for a musician these sound like pretty big obstacles to overcome. This last section is nothing more than a few thought provoking statements. Some longer, some shorter but the basis is the same. I want to challenge you to become the best version of yourself. Think differently, you know? So how do you exercise your mind?

"To live in the slums of average"

The pleasure one gets from the pursuit of pushing creative boundaries is something that goes unrivalled in the human condition. Whether it's wordplay, visual art form, music or craft, the mind craves creativity and to deprive it of that is about as logical as flailing aimlessly when trapped in the quicksand of mediocrity.

"Everyone will listen when you just STFU..."

Silence is a chapter of a book untold by most authors. Those who write it ironically live their lives in nothing but abundance of sound.

"The Power of Persuasion: Question Everything."

The art form of a question goes unnoticed by the untrained eye and ear; however my experience has shown me that single-handedly one can get their way without causing harm to relationships or themselves through this simple drill. Ask questions. Stay in control of the conversation. Don't subscribe to "fact" if you're not willing to do your due diligence to confirm words being said...

Mind - Body Co-relation: "The Body is the Mind"
- Elliot Hulse

The eagerness of childs-play is only taboo to those who are too effin' scared to live again. When one grows up he or she should only desire to be a child again.

The above quote from Elliot Hulse holds such truth and caps off this theory nicely. If you've ever felt that long, monotonous road trip turn your brain to mush and drive you to the nearest Timmy's for a double double, you know what I'm talking about. Let's think about it. You've been sitting in a van for 6 hours. No movement, no interaction. You vs. the road. Maybe some Led Zeppelin (or the Biebs again, no judgement) to pass the time, but physically you're like a bag of cement. Stiff, sore and not looking to go anywhere fast anytime soon. Trouble is, without tending to this condition, your mind will feel just as slow. So if your body feels stiff, you can bet your mind is feeling way stiff too. How much of a performer are you if your body is so rigid you can't breathe deep to get the oxygen to the important places like your brain and body? Breathe! Connect the two! Body AND Mind. You'll be amazed.

To Close...

My overall challenge to you and the one message I hope to communicate throughout these pages is that you are in complete control of your actions. We make choices. I mean, even from the top, you chose to pick this book up. After I gave you full disclosure, you made the choice to continue on all the way up to this line. And this one. Okay, now I'm just playing with you, but you get my point, right? We have the choice to do or to not do. As a musician, as a singer, as a performer... Hell, even if you're not any of those things, you're a rock star in your own right. Your kid looks up to you like you're the Mick Jagger of their world. Doesn't that mean something to you? Don't you always want to be that? Fair enough if you don't answer yes, but consider why you don't want to be the best version of yourself.

As I stated in the beginning of our relationship, I know nothing. I want to be clear about that. Nothing at all. When I approach a situation (and I'd encourage you to adopt this perspective as well) I bring with me an open mind of learning something I might not have had the opportunity to otherwise. Even if Exhibit A is an entry level, group fitness class an ignorant friend may have suggested I should partake in because it's "such a great workout!"… yet everyone there is a beginner. Hmm…

I'm still going to go to that group fitness class and learn something. I'm not above anyone.

So what I'm saying is that the key to this - all of this movement, nutrition and mindset stuff - is to remove your ego, realize there's more to it than your pride and if you take care of yourself first by admitting and addressing a possible problem, you're halfway there. In order to help you, you first have to want to help yourself. Move more, eat better and try not to sweat the small stuff. Remember, you don't have to be a rock star to start, you just have to start in order to become a rock star. Thanks for reading. Stay sweet!

The End

Acknowledgements

I don't even know where to start. I guess there are two camps that I owe a big, huge shout out to. Those who love and those who hate.

First off, all of the supporters that have helped me along the way. All you lovers out there. I mean all of you who either pushed me blindly towards that feeling of "uncomfortable" or made me check myself, and make the smart decision. Your positive influence probably saved me years putting this together and I am so grateful for your support. I'm going to list some names but I could actually write another book dedicated to everyone that has been a part of my success so please know that I love you all.

To my family: Mom, Dad - you guys have always been my biggest fans and I can't tell you how much I appreciate the way you raised all three of us. Sean, Natalie - differences aside from time to time, you know we've always got each others' backs. We should show it to each other more.

To the music community of Calgary, Alberta: you're the reason I had the crazy-ass idea to put something like this out there. From the bands I've worked with giving me the opportunity first as a musician and now as these pages are pressed, organizations like Alberta Music entrusting me as the source of all things health and wellness. To my fellow musicians and music industry professionals, weekend warriors and touring pros alike - thank you for the ongoing support and life lessons. Tanner Holthe, Jessica Marsh, Matt Blais, Noel & Candice Johnson, Lisa Anderson, The Sweets ... just to name a few of the folks that have really given me some amazing opportunities to do what I'm doing now. Thank you. Then where it all started at CHS: Scotty, Ty, K-Win… The Heist Super-Fans - Lael "Super-J", Milne, Carder, Candice. And to the Intergalactic Lovers - You guys don't even know how well timed your rock show was in Germany. I listen to Little Heavy Burdens and am immediately grateful. I hope you guys are doing well.

As far as friends go, Kevin Rae - I don't think you know that you're the reason I became a trainer, man. Without your support when I was living in Kelowna, not sure what to do with my life after that brief stint at UBCO to help me get educated and trained to become a trainer I wouldn't have had the balls to jump. Jo, thank you for letting me go from the sales side. I learned a lot, but turns out your dream was right.

Ryan Madden - you've been my best friend for as long as I can remember there through the thick and the thin and to think we'd be here when we were just rapping "It's Tricky" in the hallways of CHS is crazy. Thank you and your family for all the love and support.

Perogy - alike R-Dawg, we've basically grown up together and you've seen every side of me and always had my back. Thank you for being a rock solid force of inspiration and encouragement in all my endeavours.

Manc, we don't hang out enough 'cause you're so far away but every time we get together it's like we haven't skipped a beat. You were technically the first musician I trained with (if what you did behind the drums was considered music…) so thank you for setting me on the path! Just kidding, your knowledge of exercise, passion for people and general insight on practical life has really helped me formulate my own style of training.

Lulu - you talk funny, mate, but man did we meet at the right time. Just as this thing was taking off for me your fascination and love for experience has really helped show me that when people are determined to do, they find a way. You've also shown me first hand how positive influence, good eating and attention to one's self above all else can really change a person's outlook on life. We've been through a lot in the short time together, but you're a world class friend and one I'm very proud to call mine. You're going to do some really big things, asides from lift, bro.

To my speed skating team and friends - you guys and girls were there for me at the right time and taught me through sport that it's time to take care of your own shit. You versus the clock. No room for excuses. Get up and train. Jeff Kitura, Shannon Rempel, Donnie, Bobby, Vaughn, Jess. Thank you for your spirit in sport and great friendship. Thank you for putting up with my shit. I can't wait to get back on the ice with you.

Teddy, Ann, Danielle, Ian, Michelle & fam, Jen & Luc, Lucero, Paul & Armina, Steve, Chantal: I met all of you technically through work but you've grown into very big parts of my ongoing development and are all truly great friends. Thank you for reminding me why I am involved in the health and wellness industry and supporting me on each and every turn. And for doing those last five squats. I wish the world could see how hard you guys and gals all work. And to a new-found mentor, Wes Knight. You were my favourite Whitecap and you continue to push me to create space for the authentic soul that I am. I can't thank you more for your daily dose of inspiration, man. You're a legend! Thank you for teaching me about scarcity and abundance, jumping and being a dope soul.

I hope this book resonates with readers and shows the importance of family and friends and unconditional support. It goes without saying that there are always naysayers. For whatever reason they're there to make you stronger. If there's one thing to take away from being burned, placing trust in those who don't have your back or generally giving too much without total reciprocation it's that you will always find a way to grow and learn from that experience. The right attitude and response is key, and I'm thankful for having each individual experience that set me back at the time. To quote Canadian legend, Tom Cochrane "Life is a Highway". You bet it is, and you're the driver.

The right words or actions at the right time can motivate people crazy enough to do big things and I think my friends, family and supporters have always said the right things. Maybe not what I wanted to hear at the time but enough to empower me to fulfill my mission of inspiring others to do.

Thank you, all.

Appendices

EXTRAS

Following you will find a couple tables to help you with the movement topics discussed in the earlier sections of the book. I have included a brief description of each exercise discussed. Furthermore, please reach out to me if you would like some more assistance one-on-one with anything to do with movement, nutrition or mindset. It's what I do. Contact me for videos, pictures and the like. I'll sort you out. I know many of you will be all "dawrrr" when it comes to the descriptions. So just get at me.

www.mikeschwartz.ca

Appendix A.1

Exercise	Description
Bench Dips	• Rest your hands on a bench behind you with your feet on the floor knees bent. • Bend your elbows to lower your body. • Straighten your elbows to raise your body up then repeat.
Bicep Wall Stretch	• Standing next to a wall, place back of your hand against the wall, thumb down towards the ground • Lean towards the wall, aiming for your shoulder to touch the wall • Gently press shoulder closer to the wall until a slight stretch in the bicep is felt. Repeat on other arm.

Exercise	Description
Cat/(Cow)	• Start on your hands and knees, aligning your wrists underneath your shoulders and your knees underneath your hips. Think of the spine as a straight line connecting the crown of your head to the tailbone. This is the position of a neutral spine. Keep the neck long, as the natural extension of the spine. **Cat** • Turn the tops of your feet to the floor. • Tip your pelvis forward, tucking your tailbone like a dog would stick their tail between their legs. • Your spine will naturally round. • Brace your stomach like someone was gonna punch you. • Drop your head. **Cow** • Curl your toes under. • Tilt your pelvis back so that your butt sticks up. Think Beyonce. Twerk it. • Let this movement ripple from your tailbone up your spine so that your neck is the last thing to move. • Your belly drops down, but keep your abdominal muscles hugging your spine by bracing your stomach like someone was going to punch you. • Take your gaze up gently up toward the ceiling without cranking your neck.

Exercise	Description
Child's Pose	• Kneel on the floor. • Spread your knees as wide as your mat, keeping the tops of your feet on the floor with the big toes touching. • Bring your belly to rest between your thighs and your forehead to the floor. You can also turn your head to one side with your cheek resting on the floor. • If you choose to do that, it's a good idea to switch to the other cheek about halfway through your rest. • There are two possible arm variations. Either stretch your arms in front of you with the palms toward the floor or bring your arms back alongside your thighs with the palms facing upwards. Do whichever feels more comfortable to you. If you've been doing a lot of shoulder work, the second option feels nice. • Stay as long as you like, eventually reconnecting with the steady inhales and exhales of your breath • After your final exhale, come back up to your knees. You're done. Bravo.
Face Pulls	• Stand with your feet a comfortable distance apart. Face a cable machine and grab the two cable handles or a rope attachment with your arms at shoulder height • Slowly pull the rope back to your face, with your thumbs always staying inside so your palms face away from you • Return to the start and repeat.

Exercise	Description
Forearm Extensor Stretch	• Stand facing a bench. • Bend forward to place the backs of your hands onto the bench taking weight onto your hands with fingers facing your legs. • Straighten your arms, close your thumbs to your fingers and attempt to lift your knuckles off the bench. • Hold the stretch then relax.
Forearm Flexor Stretch	• Stand facing a bench. • Bend forward to place your palms onto the bench taking weight onto your hands with fingers pointed back to your body. • Press your palms into the bench while lifting your fingers. • Hold the stretch then relax.
Horse Stance, Dynamic	• Kneel on all fours, place your hands directly underneath your shoulders and knees under your hips. • Legs should be parallel and elbows tucked back towards your thighs, fingers facing forward. • Inhale while raising your right arm up and out to a 45 °angle also lifting your leg up and back behind you as high as you can without your pelvis swaying to the side. • Exhale and tuck your knee and elbow under your torso so your elbow goes past your knee.

Exercise	Description
Inchworm/Hand Walkout	• Stand with feet a comfortable distance apart. • Bend forward from the hips placing your hands on the ground. • Slowly walk your hands out in front of you while keeping your legs straight until you're fully extended, face down hands and toes touching the ground • Contract your abs, brace your abs like you're getting punched and go only as far as you comfortably can. • Walk your hands back the same way you walked them out, straight-legged
McKenzie Press Up	• Lie on the floor face down with your hands just outside the top of your shoulders. • Inhale as you push yourself up keeping your pelvis on the floor relaxing your back and butt. • Exhale as you lower.
Medicine Ball (MB) Russian Twist	• Lie on your back with arms out at shoulder height, palms up with your hips and knees bent to 90°with a medicine ball held between your knees. • Drawing your belly button inwards twist your trunk to the side to lower your legs and the ball towards the floor then use your abdominals to twist your lower body back to the start. • Lower to the opposite side and repeat performing a twisting motion from one side to the other.

Exercise	Description
Modified Reverse Grip Push Up	• Lie face down, hands at a comfortable width at shoulder height. Rotate hands back so your fingers are pointing away and outside your body, not up towards your head • Take a deep breath and brace your abs. Exhale through pursed lips pushing yourself up to a plank position keeping your head and spine in alignment. • Inhale as you lower back to the ground. • Repeat for the prescribed number of reps and gradually increase your hands rotation so eventually your thumbs are pointing away from you body, fingers pointing towards your toes.
Neck Rolls	• Let your head drop down naturally as you exhale. • Rotate it around slowly letting it follow your natural range of motion. Inhale as you begin moving to the side and back. • Spend extra time in tight zones: imagine that you are breathing through the tight muscles.
Pec Major/Minor Wall Stretch	• Stand facing a wall. • Raise one arm up and place your hand and forearm against the wall at about 90° • Step forward moving your body in towards the wall to the point where you feel a comfortable stretch across your chest.

Exercise	Description
Quadruped Shoulder Twister	• Kneel on all fours with good spine alignment horizontal to floor, keep elbows bent. • Drawing your belly button in towards your spine take one arm out to the side to shoulder height with your elbow bent to 90° twisting your elbow and shoulders up towards the sky. • Hold for the prescribed time, perform on the opposite side, then repeat.
Scap/Stability Push Up	• Hands and knees on the floor in a kneeling push up position. • Maintaining a neutral spine and straight arms lower your chest towards the floor, squeeze your shoulder blades together. • Push with straight arms to raise your chest up between your shoulder blades as high as possible and repeat.
Shoulder Clocks	• Lie down on your side with your knees bent. Your bottom arm should hold your head up and your top arm should rest on your side • Visualize that your shoulder is in the middle of a clock. • Elevate your shoulder toward your ear (12 clock) then roll your shoulder forwards around the clock. Inhale from 12-6 and exhale from 6-12. • Repeat in the opposite direction keeping your body relaxed.

Exercise	Description
"Shoulder Check" Cobra	• Lie face down with your arms at your sides. • As you inhale pick your chest up off the floor with the neck in neutral alignment simultaneously squeezing your shoulder blades together and rotating your arms out so the palms face away from your body. Now, turn your head as if to "shoulder check" off to the right side, then the left. • You should feel the muscles between your shoulder blades doing the work. If you feel stress in your low back squeeze your bum prior to lifting your torso. • Hold until you need to breathe out and exhale as you lower.
Supine Single Leg Glute Stretch	• Lie on your back on the floor • Cross your leg placing your ankle on your opposite knee. Hold your knee and ankle. • Pull with your arms and push with your lower leg to move your crossed leg towards your chest to the point that you feel a comfortable stretch in your glute. • Hold the stretch then repeat on the other side.

Exercise	Description
Stationary Lunge	• Take a split stance so that your back thigh and front shin are perpendicular to the ground when you lower down. Brace your abs as if you were going to be punched. • Keeping good posture, lower to the point where your back knee just touches the ground. • Come back up. Your front shin should stay perpendicular with the ground on the lowering and rising phase of the movement.
Sub-Occipital Stretch	• Sit on a bench, place one hand on your chin and one hand on the back of your head. • Gently tuck your chin to stretch the back of your neck.
Supermans	• Lie face down, lift both arms and legs off the ground so they are about the same height off the ground • Your thumbs should be facing up and your arms around 45° from your head. • Lower and repeat for the prescribed number of reps.
Supine Hip Raise	• Lie face up, bend your knees and plant you feet close to your bum • Brace your abdomen as if you were to be punched and slowly raise your hips up to the sky, squeezing your bum and keeping your abs braced. Inhale as you push your hips to the sky, exhale as you lower them • Repeat for the prescribed number of reps.

Exercise	Description
Supine Knee Drop	• Lie on your back with your knees bent and feet together on the floor, spaced about a foot away from your bum. Play around with the position. Make it comfy. • Let your legs drop gently to one side and then the other. Inhale as they drop, exhale as you pick them back up
Swiss Ball (SB) Lat Stretch	• Kneel with a Swiss ball in front of you. Place both forearms on the ball. • Push your hips backwards to your feet, then drop your head between your extended arms until you feel a comfortable stretch down your arms and back.
Swiss Ball (SB) Lower Body Rotation	• Lie on your back with your thighs vertical and knees bent to 90°, place a Swiss ball between your feet and keep your arms out at shoulder height, palms up. • Brace your abs and twist to lower your thighs to the floor. • Slowly return to the start and repeat twisting to each side.
Trapezius Lateral Stretch	• Sit on a bench, reach down and grab a hold of the bench to anchor your shoulder. • Drop your head down, then bend it to the side and rotate slightly towards the anchored shoulder.

Exercise	Description
Tricep Wall Stretch	• Stand parallel to a wall. • Reach up as far as possible with your right arm rising onto your toes and place your elbow against the wall. • Lower your body to standing as you bend your right elbow to reach behind your back. • Keeping your neck in neutral, rotate your wrist in each direction to vary the stretch and check for which position is tightest. • Hold the stretch in the position of tightness contracting your biceps to increase the stretch. • Relax then repeat on the other side
Wag the Tail	• Kneel on all fours with your hips over your knees, shoulders over your wrists. • Contract your abs and gently let your hips fall towards the ground towards one side. • Bring yourself back up and repeat towards the other side.
Waiter's Bow	• Stand with your feet parallel and close together. Keeping your legs straight, push your bum back until you have an arch in your low back, like a waiter would serve a fancy glass of chardonnay. • Bend forward from the hips holding the arch in your low back until you feel a comfortable stretch in the hamstrings.

Exercise	Description
Wall Angel/Scarecrow	• Stand upright with your back against a wall, take your feet out about a foot away from the wall (sometimes further if your back doesn't flatten out) • Brace your abs and press your back, crown of your head and hips tight against the wall. • Raise your arms out up to shoulder height while trying to keep your back, hips, shoulders, arms and wrists against the wall. • Slowly drop your hands to your side, returning to the start position and repeat.
Windshield Wipers	• Lie down on your back with your arms out at shoulder height (palms up); your thighs vertical and knees bent to 90° (to start. Eventually you will have the strength to keep your legs straight) • Brace your abs and let your legs slowly lower to the floor together on one side then tighten your abs to pick the legs back up. • Lower to the opposite side and repeat performing a twisting motion from one side to the other. Like a windshield wiper on an old car.

Appendix A.2

EXERCISE VARIABLES

Variable	Definition
Sets	This is how many groups of the drill you should perform.
Repetitions	This is how many consecutive times you should perform the drill
Intensity	This is how heavy the load is. 95% MAX means 95% of your maximum effort. (Something you'll likely never touch in the early stages) Something more common would be BW (bodyweight), or RM - (Rep Max) where you perform the exercise using only your own body weight or perform the exercise with a weight that causes you to fatigue at the prescribed number of repetitions.
Tempo	How fast you move during the motion. Can be "slow", "breathing", "fast" etc, or written out in seconds ie. 303 - which means 3 seconds going into the motion, no pause at the bottom and then 3 seconds back to the start of the motion.
Rest	How much time you must wait before starting things back up for the next set.

References

If you're interested in learning more about the specific references I uhh… make reference to… take a peek below:

Precision Nutrition Certification Manual 2nd Edition: The Essentials of Sport and Exercise Nutrition

http://firstendurance.com/anti-inflammatory-foods/

http://chekinstitute.com/blog/you-just-cant-cheat-nature-circadian-rhythms-and-your-hormones/

http://www.nature.com/nm/journal/v1/n10/full/nm1095-1009.html

http://www.precisionnutrition.com/encyclopedia/food/sodium/

(other indirect references may exist and your best bet if you wanna find out what the eff I'm talking about is to just contact me directly!)

www.ingramcontent.com/pod-product-compliance
Lightning Source LLC
Chambersburg PA
CBHW030414290526
45785CB00004B/1994